CIRCADIA
HEART R
PRESSURE

BY

Garima Bharti

ACKNOWLEDGEMENT

This thesis is the culmination of my journey of PhD which was just like climbing a high peak step by step accompanied with encouragement, hardship, trust, and frustration. When I found myself at top experiencing the feeling of fulfillment, I realized that only my name will appear on the cover of this dissertation but inevitable support of many people in this journey will remain dormant those have contributed to accomplish this huge task. Therefore, through this acknowledgement I want to give the due credit to all those people.

At this moment of accomplishment words are inadequate to express my gratitude to my guide respected **Dr. Ajit Pal Singh**, Professor & HOD, Department of Anatomy and co- guide **Dr. Pankaj Kumar**, Professor & HOD, Department of Biochemistry, HDCH, Sundernagar, (H.P) for their constant encouragement, affectionate guidance,

moral support and constructive criticism in this work. I am very grateful to respected **Dr. Pankaj Soni**, medical Tutor specialist, Department of Anatomy, Shri Lal Bahadur Shastri GMCH, Mandi, (H.P) for helping me in my work. I would also like to thanks **Dr. Indu Bansal** (HOD), Department of Physiology, for her help & valuable guidance.

Finally, I want to express my gratitude to my father **Er. Ramesh Chand Bharti**, my Mother **Mrs. Kusum Bharti** & brother Viresh for their endless love, support and Blessings, without them I could not accomplish this task. Moreover, I am thankful to my Husband, Advocate **Mr. Deepak Sehgal** without his consistent encouragement, faith and liberal attitude towards me, inspired me to achieve my goal with determination. I would also like to thanks Mrs. Divya (Anatomy) & Mr. Raj Sharma (med. chemistry) for their valuable suggestions. Further, I am also thankful to all my family members for the selfless love, care and sacrifice to shape my life.

Above all, I thank the Almighty for giving me the strength and patience to work through for all these years so that today I could live a life of respect, integrity and prestige in the society.

Garima Bharti

LIST OF CONTENTS

LIST OF TABLES

LIST OF FIGURES

LIST OF ABBREVIATIONS

A: Amplitude

AA: African Americans

ABPM: Ambulatory Blood Pressure Monitor

ANOVA: Analysis of Variance

BMI: Body Mass index

BP: Blood Pressure

BPV: Blood Pressure Variability

BSA: Body Surface Area

CHD: Coronary Heart Disease

CR: Circadian Rhythms

CTS: Circadian Timing System

CVD: Cardiovascular Diseases

D: Dipper

DBP: Diastolic Blood Pressure

df: Degree of freedom

DMRT: Duncan's Multiple Range test

DP: Double Product

EAS: European Americans

ED: Extreme Dipper

F: Statistic

HR: Heart Rate

HRV: Heart Rate Variability

LD: Light/Dark
M: Mesor

MAP: Mean Arterial Pressure

MBPS: Morning Blood Pressure Surge

ND: Non Dipper

NS: Not Significant

PP: Pulse Pressure

RD: Rhythm Detection

RDR: Rhythmic Detection Ratio

ROM: Read only Memory

S: Significant

SBP: Systolic Blood Pressure

SPPC: Statistical Package for the Social Sciences t:

Prominent time

Ø: Aerophase or Peak

Z: Prominent Period

ABSTRACT

Blood pressure variability (BPV) is one of the major risk factors for several types of cardiovascular diseases (CVDs). This review focuses on behavioral aspects of circadian rhythms of both males & females. It is valuable, therefore, to demonstrate the circadian variability in systolic blood pressure (SBP), diastolic blood pressure (DBP) and Heart Rate (HR) in both males as well as female subjects with special reference to age, sex, work type & dipping patterns. In our findings, we aimed to clarify the fluctuations among men & women. A total of 300 voluntarily participated in the study. All subjects wore an Ambulatory Blood Pressure Monitor

SBP, DBP and HR were measured every 20 and 40 minutes. In addition, double product (DP) and mean arterial pressure (MAP) were also documented. Data were analyzed using A&D, Cosinor and Spectra software. A statistically significant Circadian rhythm was validated in all studied components, with respect to Age, Sex, type of work & dipping pattern. Additionally, significant differences for the circadian Mesors, Amplitude, Acrophase of SBP, DBP, HR, DP and MAP were also noticed. Results show that, as the age increases Mesor of SBP, DBP& MAP increases in males but in case of females, Amplitude of SBP was more. In males dipping was less than females. Diurnal SBP, DBP, MAP were higher in extreme Dippers whereas nocturnal values were higher in non dippers. We also proved that in subjects with medications had more non dipping pattern. In hypertensive subjects without medications & non dipper the rhythm detection ratio was low particularly in SBP, MAP.

On the basis of our findings we can summarized that variability in BP may be related to Age, Sex & type of work to some extent.

Keywords: ABPM; Blood Pressure; Heart Rate; Circadian Rhythm; Double Product; Mean Arterial Pressure.

CHAPTER-I

INTRODUCTION

All the undeveloped nations Hypertension may be a frequent alarm, irrespective of their stage of health alteration. Particularly it"s a hazardous component for cardiac arrest, ischemic stroke, and kidney dysfunction is Hypertension. Occurrence of hypertension is different in each developed as well as undeveloped nations. Reported by Singh *et al.*, 2000 stroke and prevalence of hypertension is a cause of rapid increase in mortality in developing countries of Asia. Studies conducted between 1980 and 2003 Kearney *et al.*, 2004 shows the occurrence of hypertension has attenuated in advanced countries, but inflated in underdeveloped countries. There is no notable difference in the mean incidence, alertness, cure and management of Blood Pressure between advanced and undeveloped nations, but there is an associate degree of occurrence through males in advanced countries Pereira *et al.*, 2009. In addition, they came to the conclusion that the occurrence, alertness, cure, and management of Blood pressure in undeveloped nations are coming closer to those in advanced nations. It affects large number of population and increasing tendency in the occurrences of High BP and Coronary Heart Failure (CHF) which has been announced in our nation (Gopinath *et al.*, 1994; Pais *et al.*, 1996; Gupta, 2004; Kusuma *et al.*, 2004; Rao *et al.*, 2011. In India, among urban areas the occurrence of Blood Pressure was expected higher as compared to the rural population (Kusuma *et al.*, 2004; Kusuma and Das, 2008).

One of the most challenging and exciting area in present day science and medicine is study of circadian rhythm. Rhythm means series of events which repeat themselves in organized manner. It is defined as circadian period which ranges in between 20-28 hours. Less than this called ultradian and longer then this period infradian. Helberg introduced it to describe those biorhythms which are for around 24 hours. From surrounding impact, i.e., dissimilarity in bodily and intellectual activity and tension during day to day activity vs. dark sleep, and the stage relations of a several endogenic biorhythms, the 24-hrs changes in CV system physiology and physiopathology appears.

Human beings make clear circadian rhythm in different behavioral and Physiological variables, irrespective of enzyme actions, rest-activity, bodily responses, hormones production and body temperature (Redfern and Lemmer, 1997). This variable shows twenty hours rhythms as far as they persist coordinated within outer circadian pattern. Nevertheless, in both cases, these rhythms freely move and indicate periods very approximate to 24 hours. The dissimilarity around sleeping & waking Systolic BP measures and Diastolic BP measures were more. Formerly proclaimed that during daily routine besides the general BP varies widely rises in persons with high BP, but also the variations are less as compared to Normal blood pressure individuals (Mancia *et al.*, 1983, 1997, 2003).

Over a 24-hours period Blood pressure is not stable, it varies. Blood pressure fluctuates daily in answer to mental and physical activities and show signs of reproducible patterns of climax and depression. Other multi-frequency rhythms apart from circadian rhythms in humans, specifically Circannual rhythms, Circaseptan rhythms and Circasemiseptan rhythms were enumerated from BP as well as pulse

Rate (Rawson *et al.*, 2000). In relation to these rhythms, in Normotensive and Hypertensive humans biorhythms in Pressure level has already studied which belongs to the tepid climates of Earth (Gonzalez *et al.*, 2002; Cornélissen *et al.*, 2003; Halberg *et al.*, 2004). Union is lacking behind concerning intrinsic character of arterial Pressure pattern. However, in both men & women, arterial Pressure drops in the course of sleeping time and remains high during the waking time with a significantly flow during sunrise (Redon, 2004). Hypertensive subjects whose Arterial Pressure remains elevated during dark time (non-dippers) are at high chances for CVS illness as compared to dippers (Verdecchia *et al.*, 1996). Injury to CNS, CVS and Renal is much larger in High BP non-dippers; the last mentioned also offer bad diagnosis for CVS events as diierentiated to dippers (Shimada *et al.*, 1992; O"Brien *et al.*, 1988; Verdecchia *et al.*, 1990, 1994; Imai *et al.*, 1996; Kobrin *et al.*, 1984).

Significance of ABPM has been expanded for the detection of high BP. It is helpful for supplying an average arterial pressure during day time / night time and the normal range of Ambulatory BPM has been overall less than fundamental BP values (Imai *et al.*, 1996). One time inspection of pressure level is not trustworthy for detecting high BP.

The pressure level changeability pattern varies in infected and high blood pressure persons. Circadian and Circaseptan rhythms (Rawson *et al.*, 2000) studied in Pressure level and Pulse rate in a mentally stressed person & the Circaseptan elements of these variations should be assessed widely if pineal organ of endocrine gland is present in this processed underlying mental disease. Yet, the BP changeability may play an important role in mental illness in humans. It is said that unexpected coronary failure, coronary thrombosis, Heart arrest, ventricular arrhythmias, cardiopulmonary arrest, Heart attack, cerebro-vascular all these occurs in the morning when blood pressure increases unexpectedly (Redon, 2004). The onset of indications of most of the heart diseases is dependent upon time.

The changeability in arterial pressure exist in normal person with accordance to sex, life span, & its origin describes elevated level of Mesor, descending of amplitude and development in Peak of systolic SBP as well as diastole BP with growing age (Driziene *et al.*, 2008).It has been suggested that the biorhythm of pressure level should be assessed in accordance to Gender, Age and race-matched reference values (Driziene *et al.*, 2008).

Several ranges of work which is associated with pulse rate variability beside various physio-pathologic situations, as well as exaggerated chances of death (Kleiger *et al.*, 1987). The 2 necessary factors particularly span and sex, modifying the pulse rate of normal individualls (Umetani *et al.*, 1998).Pulse rate variability was seen diminished with the development moving on (O"Brien *et al.,* 1986; Ori *et al.*, 1992; Umetani *et al.*, 1998). Though, the relationship among HRV and sex is significantly arguable; whereas pulse rate was higher in women as compared to men (Gowan *et al.*, 1995; Huikuri *et al.*, 1996), the alternatives have conjointly delineating (Rich *et al.*, 1988; Van Hoogenhuyze *et al.*, 1991).

In addition, nocturnal dropping in vital sign may be a traditional development. Nevertheless, among Normotensive individuals this fall is the main sign throughout sleeping time doesn't forever occur (Larochelle, 2002). Human subjects are often categorized into dippers, non-dippers, extreme dippers and risers on the premise of the nocturnal dipping in vital sign. In dippers, vital sign stated a decline of concerning 10- 20% throughout sleeping hours; whereas in non-dippers it's solely concerning 0-10% (Thomas *et al.*, 2006). The intense Dippers indicate quite two hundredth dipping and also the risers register increased Pressure level throughout sleeping pattern. The development of night time dipping in vital sign has predictive importance for vessel mortality, cardiac arrest and advancement to excretion of urinary albumin in Type-1 or 2 polygenic diseases (Pistrosch *et al.*, 2007).

Hajjar *et al.,* 2010 steered about nighttime lowering BP ought to acquire within the advanced analysis of people who were having chance of neural structure sickness. Additionally, investigations on Diurnal-Nocturnal variations in Blood Pressure are an extra necessary space for analysis. Superabundant reports are out there that has investigated Diurnal-Nocturnal alternations in Blood Pressure in Normal individual and persons full of numerous infections (Broadhurst *et al.*, 1990; Boggia *et al.*, 2007). Variations on daytime and dark vital sign have conjointly been analyzed with relation to Age, Gender, and quality (Broadhurst *et al.*, 1990; Wang *et al.*, 2006, 2009). Foreboding importance of day against dark vital sign has been inspected (Palatini *et al.*, 1992; Kikuya *et al.*, 2006; Boggia *et al.*, 2007; Thijs *et al.*, 2007). It's been incontestable that dark Blood Pressure ranges are a lot of dependable forecaster for the day time Blood Pressure variations (Eguchi *et al.*, 2009). The Impact of psycho-emotional & bodily strain might weakens the prophetic worth of diurnal Blood Pressure, whereas more consistency ensuing from sleeping might facilitates to illustrate correlation with night Blood Pressure (Khirmanov and Tiurina, 2002). Boggia *et al.*, 2007 guided regarding the exactness of the diurnal & nocturnal Blood Pressure which rely on the top points below findings. The essential sign variability in day-night was conjointly seen related to nocturnal vital sign, drop in Normal and High BP persons (Verdecchia *et al.*, 1994). Twenty four hours variation and day time / dark variations in BP are often monitored victimization the non-invasive device; mobile vital sign monitor (ABPM). Within department of vital sign analysis, twenty four apparatus is taken into account which is a helpful diving device in Hypertensive subjects as well as Normotensive individuals. Disparity in time unit cycle i.e. nocturnal dipping, and day time / dark variations in vital sign can't be calculated on the premise of single spot examination. For that reason, in recent times to induce higher results, to enhance the designation and treatment of high blood pressure and vessel diseases clinicians deem mobile vital sign observance. As per data available, in the Asian countries, studies on circadian rhythms in human vital sign and rate victimization Ambulatory Blood Pressure Monitoring aren't enough. Additionally, studies on variations in daytime and dark BP are negligible.

Increased occurrence of BP in Asia has been reported in recent time, which is an alarming situation and is presumed with the abnormality in Blood Pressure. Therefore the present study "circadian variations of heart rate and blood pressure in Normotensive and Hypertensive North Indians" will definitely helpful for the Govt. for nation-wide programs.

NEED OF STUDY

In modern period it"s been shocking spread regarding occurrence of High BP and Coronary heart diseases (CHD) in our country. It"s supposed that the circumstances should be assigned to associated occurrence of irregularity in pressure level variables. Unexpectedly, data on pressure level variability from Chronobiological part is very less in the nation. Thus, we suggest that there should be a various initiative Schemes be established for studying BPV in India including both normal and high BP individuals. Our aim is, the outcomes acquired & described in this work will give useful information to research-based section on BPV in human population of India. Additionally, a comparison between normal & high BP persons of BPV might contribute to the present work. End result of our work may be beneficial in: (i) creating the standard measurements of BP and Pulse Rate in accordance to sex & age, (ii) estimating the respective role of High BP,(iii) describing proposals for controlling several Coronary Heart diseases in our nation.

AIMS AND OBJECTIVES

1. To study and documentation of the circadian variations of Heart Rate & BP in normal human subjects from Panchkula, using ABPM.
2. To study changes in the sequences of circadian variations of HR & BP in hypertensive humans.
3. To compare the present findings with available literature.

CHAPTER-II

REVIEW OF LITERATURE

Among the foremost substantial options of the globe during which we tend to survive is the biological day-night process. This "biological clock," induces the living creatures to initiate & gear up alterations in our surroundings during day & dark, inevitable making sure that the living creatures work properly at the correct time. The mechanism conjointly gives intrinsic time based company with making clear intrinsic alterations happened in systematic manner. Researchers began finding out biological rhythms or so sixty years past. Temporal organization"s revelations in biomes square measure called as „Biological Rhythms" that square measure present among living organisms. Circadian rhythm is well know term in science. It is a natural process, which keeps sleep-wake cycle regulating and also repeats roughly every 24 hours.

Halberg, 1959 coiled of the terms "Circadian" & "chronobiology" (Halberg, 1969). Chronomedicine may be a different space of chronobiology, which aims to boost the present and forms new strategies of bar, new ways signs of treatment of assorted abnormality on the premise of the chronobiological knowledge. The Chronomedicine has an objective to recognize common and particular forms of biological clock violation which is consequent to diseased form and thus develops techniques for amendments in humans.

Kleitman, 1963 was the first to check the individuals unit of time rhythms. In 1938, he demonstrated a practical on 2 subjects deep beneath the cave.

Halberg *et al.*, 1972 introduced the field that equitably adjudge & explore procedure of time formed; together with swingy abstract of existence is termed as "Chronobiology".

Brown, 1972 explicit Biological periodicity is also responsible in behavior as well as other mutating acceptance of an individual to all the elements which include the habitat and narcotics etc. The biological periodicity could also be of variable period starting from a friction of seconds to years.

Pittendrigh and Daan, 1976 presented conceptual knowledge regarding operation of the unit of time clock formed from scientist who worked on flies.

7

Chronotherapeutics is the most developed part of Chronomedicine, and its main object is to develop the strategies to effects the illness methods by taking into considerations the individual Chronobiological features of the subjects.

Jurgen Aschoff, Franz Halberg and Colin Pittendrigh dispended the existence of endogenous unit of time clock. Aschoff *et al.*, 1967; Aschoff and Wever, 1976) discovered and interpretated the development of "spontaneous internal desynchronization" & was an actuation in unit of time physiology for many years.

Abnormal biological time of pressure level is prone to multiplied hazards of disorders i.e. issues related to sleeping patterns, metabolic syndrome, CVDs and cancerous growth. Besides this, Blood Pressure level watching of twenty four (24 hrs.), methods for analyzing the unusual form of low BP level, over night is getting least doctors attentiveness. Time unit (Circadian) rhythms are known to have an effect on body functions which are controlled by the hypothalamus and Cerebral Cortex.

Desir *et al.*, 1981 declared that tiredness forms a movement in behavioral, bodily & secretion biorhythms in individuals and it"s of nice interest to unit of time researchers because of fast arrangement and desire for later re-mounting of the unit of time management. Persons moving towards distinct geographical areas ought to be entrained to the new LD cycle.

Muller *et al.*, 1985; Rocco *et al.*, 1987 thought of numerous announced, the reoccurrence of coronary infraction peaks around six in the morning & evening and noon and McFadden, 1988 thought of individual having respiratory disorder suffer most current attack at dark time.

Van Cauter, 1989 advised that the secretions of many hormones conjointly occur during cyclic fashion. For instance, the regular flow of lactogen and somatotropin gets enhanced while sleeping (Van Cauter, 1987).

Harshfield *et al.*, 1989 and Suzuki *et al.*, 1993 stated the variations of biorhythm elements of Pressure level has been elevated in normal individuals in relation to their age, sex. On the other side quality High pressure may be a general

disorder in each specified underdeveloped nations. Biological time in pressure level was seen in persons having long lasting pressure issues along with night time pressure dropping is also elevated in few patients.

Verdacchia *et al.*, 1990 presented that High Blood Pressure Patients without night BP fall (non-Dipper) were more prone to extreme organs damages than whose Blood Pressure falls (Dipper) throughout the night.

Rawson *et al.*, 2000 has been considerable discussing concerning endogenic behavior of Pressure level bio rhythm. However, in individuals, throughout sleep BP drops significantly and during waking period remains elevated with a significantly flow in first brightening hours. The attributes of BP pattern are far formed to change in sick people. Extreme day to day peak is treated as CHAT i.e. circadian hyper amplitude–tension. It has been connected with the most important far formed risk of cerebral anemia disease and additionally with a high threat for Heart attack, Peripheral nervous system diseased and loss of vision.

Redwine *et al.*, 2000 determined that a non regulation of the sleeping awakening cyclic process harm sum total of current blood cells and therefore ensuring immunity alterations forms several bad fitness consequences. These inflaming reactants are involved for major cause in diseases together with fatness, diabetes, carcinoma, neuro degenerative & vas complications (Sarkisian *et al.*, 2017).

Lambert *et al.*, 2001 demonstrated fluctuation of Blood Pressure occurs in 24- hours amount and show duplicable patterns of climax concerning intellectual & bodily performance. Presently scientists are showing their curiosity within the review of Secular Corporation within the BP profile. Today in modern world the researchers have confidence on ABPM so that we can upgrade the detection of disease and medical curing BP and CHD. ABPM may be a instrument, that generates BP values in movable & sleeping state.

Duffy *et al.*, 2001 demonstrated the time unit series adjusts the variations in varied execution, Endocrine pattern, functioning, sleeping time etc. The exciting thing

of biorhythms is, though during lack of extrinsic stimulant, nearly twenty four hrs biorhythms are sustained (Czeisler and Gooley, 2007).

Seo and Oh 2002 biological time in BP has been broadly speaking studies in normotensive and hypertensive subjects except from day to day rhythms, different range of density biorhythms, specifically Circaseptan Circasemiseptan as well as Circannual has additionally been delineated for Normal and High BP patients.

Al-Hazimi *et al.*, 2002 instructed that severe variation in Pulse Rate is usually related to disorders. Calculations of Pulse Rate Variations are progressively worked as indication of internal organ involuntary work, diabetes mellitus pathology as well as alternative disorders.

Mokdad *et al.*, 2004 Highlighted the origin of death in cultured classes, that have transferred from contagious or spreadable to non-contagious or non-spreadable long lasting illness like CVS, High BP, high glucose level, Carcinoma, Arterial Blood vessel sickness disease and diseases of Chronic inflammation.

Sahna *et al.*, 2005 higher likelihood of developing cardiopathy or internal organ mortality established in persons having low nightly condensed melatonin.

Schwartzkopff *et al.*, 2005 advised that Pressure level measurement through the assistance of Ambulatory device without break for twenty four hrs period might give a helpful result.

Boggia *et al.*, 2007 evaluated that Blood Pressure Variability (BPV) could be complicated development. Variations in pressure level is one in every of the identified threat for various forms of heart disorders. Further, day/night fluctuations in Pressure level in Normal healthy people and individuals moving through numerous disorders that have been assessed generally.

Prasai *et al.*, 2008 demonstrated that Coronary heart diseases are the foremost vital reason of death in advanced nations imputed by circadian disruption.

Brotman *et al.*, 2008 explained that getting dark (nightly) decreases in Pressure level is the most prime feature of unit of time in physically fit persons. Prophecy importance of nightly pressure level dropping has previously demonstrated heart blockage, CHD, and development of micro proteinuria in both diabetic types.

Murray *et al.*, 2009 mentioned the unit of time organization adjusts award encouragement. Present composition on award encouragement gives almost negligible awareness to the actual findings that pays possibility of the climate differs extremely with the LD cyclic manner.

Kabutoya *et al.*, 2010 dictated increase within the threat of vessels disorders along with the flow of amount drops in nighttime pressure level (non-dipping) & Pulse Rate. On other side, individual claiming for pattern of pressure level wherever the center level doesn"t decreases in the dark, have a poorer cardiovascular prognosis.

M.C. Acelajado *et al.*, 2012 dispended a study which includes a group thirty eight patients with AH. Out of which 13 patients were dippers and half dozen - darkness pickers, remaining subjects were irregular to teams of sunrise and sunset uptake.The variability in Blood Pressure of Hypertensive Patient is the prime risk factor of Heart Diseases, especially in stroke cases. Forecast is upsetting & is formed on plain clinical verification. Elevated pressure level is, primarily, a threatening issue for coronary conditions so there is no question regarding this very fact that Heart failures is inevitable causes of death all over the world. Nowadays, India is one of the leading countries in the incidences related to high BP and various Heart disorders amongst resident. Moreover, lack of awareness regarding blood pressure variability on human population is the reason for such incidence in the Indian sub-continent. Hence, it is imperative to lead a common mass programmes all over to review the variability of BP in every healthy & High BP Patients.

Hermida *et al.*, 2013 rumored that taking any high Blood Pressure medicines during bedtime, will cut back pressure level throughout sleeping hrs and produce back the traditional pattern of BP in few patients.

Dixit and Singh, 2013 advised that the secretions of many hormones conjointly occur during cyclic fashion. For instance, the regular flow of lactogen and somatotropin gets enhanced while sleeping.

Qian and Scheer, 2016 explained that besides, day to day interruptions in living beings might elevate diabetes threat through inflaming process which is free from sleep loss, hatching to desend insulin reactivity without balancing elevated insulin production.

Among numerous rhythms in soma, sleeping/awakening cycle is probably the foremost raw indication of unit time patterns. Different rhythms management a lot of the human body"s traditional functions, as well as performance, behavior, endocrine secretions, heartbeat, and vital sign.

ABPM methodology conjointly permits to spot subjects with early morning high Blood Pressure and morning BP surge (MBPS). In first two hours after waking up, high Blood Pressure is primarily increased. There"s not any accord on the MBPS illumination, maximum investigators make utilization of strategy projected by Kario *et al.* The scientists calculated MBPS in two forms: the increase in Blood Pressure throughout sleeping, therefore known as «sleeptrough MBPS», outlined because the distinction between the early morning BP (average BP throughout the prior 2 hours when rousing) & therefore lowest night time average BP (average of 3 measurements - the least nocturnal value + both measurements instantly prior & afterwards); and the elevated Blood Pressure before rising - reawakening MBPS, demarcated due to distinction among sunrise and before waking up BP (average BP two hrs prior to waking up).

CHAPTER-III

MATERIAL AND METHODS

The current work was done in Panchkula, state of Haryana. A total number of 300 subjects were included and divided in different categories Normotensive and Hypertensive groups (with or without medicine).

Ethical clearance was taken from Desh Bhagat University, Punjab (India). Informed consent to conduct the survey "Circadian variations of Heart Rate and Blood Pressure in Normotensive and Hypertensive North Indians" was also taken before the study.

This work entitled as, "Circadian variations of Heart Rate and Blood Pressure in Normotensive and Hypertensive North Indians" and was divided into following stages.

The first stage includes assessment of work that was performed on variations of Pressure level and Pulse Rate in Normal and High Blood pressure subjects.

The second stage was concerned with Circadian Variations in Pressure Level and Pulse Rate in normal individuals, who were from Panchkula region in the state of Haryana in accordance to Age, sex and kind of Work.

The third stage consists of the day to day fluctuations in Pressure Level and Pulse Rate in High Blood Pressure subjects.

The available data was studied, analyzed, documented & compared with other studies to find out any variations.

INCLUSIVE CRITERIA

Subjects who were willing to take part in our work were

included. **EXCLUSIVE CRITERIA**

1. Subjects not willing to participate.
2. School going students, children who were below 18 yrs.
3. All subjects with serious complications like cancer, malignancy, mentally

retarded etc were exempted.

INSTRUMENT USED

ABPM: Ambulatory Blood Pressure Monitor is an instrument used during this study. The device is applied to measure Blood Pressure (BP). It almost stores three hundred records of common user and three hundred fifty data of ABP. Each data contains complete components of BP, Error message and also stores numbers. This instrument includes 2.4 inch color LCD. It unified data noticed functions and an exhibit function which includes data review, facts list, Blood Pressure data style chart, the present clock timing, detailed information, and also buzzer. Person can switch on/off the LCD. There is sound and light alarm beeping with red light appearing to induce battery dropping. Sound beeps when the recorded number result rises .The person can switch on/ off the buzzer if he wants to.

Atop of instrument the cuff opening is located. Multi functions can be done with the help of PC software, and the stored data can also be shifted to computer.

PROCESS

Firstly we start ABPM by turning it on. It shows flash once, which indicates that boot-band, is ready. Then sensor is connected between the Monitor and the patient.

In common user system, the apparatus will turn off LCD when no button is pushed down and turns into constant mode, if there is no function performed then also the gadget will itself turn off. During low power, battery progress bar is empty, and then red indicator flashes with buzzer.

· In the Main Interface:

At the left top of the screen, alarm switches exhibits. User bar displays the common user's data record with current patient type. On the middle top of the screen, Current date and time (seconds) is displayed.

1. System is switched on.
2. BP cuff is applied to subject‟s upper forelimb.
3. Then cuff is connected to the air hose. The arm must be at patient's heart level.

4. Appropriately mode is adopted.

5. Switch is pressed and readings are measured.

LIMITATIONS OF MEASUREMENTS

The oscillometric measurement has some limitations also

- Patient Movement: Patient should be still without any movements, like shaking, palpitations, jerkings etc. These movements may obstruct with the spotting of the Arterial Pulses, prolonged time.
- Cardiac Arrhythmia's: Irregular Heartbeat Measurements in case of Cardiac Arrhythmia, prolonged time.
- Heart-lung Machine: Patient, if connected to a heart-lung machine, measurement is not possible.
- Pressure Changes: Blood Pressure of a patient, if fluctuates quickly over the period of time, no assessments done.
- Shock: During severe shock or Hypothermia, recordings will be false, so person is advised to sit still.
- HR Extremes: Recordings can"t be done if HR is less than 40 beats per min and more than 240 beats per min.

INSTALLING SOFTWARE

1. Firstly we placed CD ROM (programmable read-only memory) on that particular section, and then CD ROM is played.

2. CD in reader is played and instructions are followed when they are displayed on particular LCD; or we can take the following installing directions: 1. Windows Explorer is opened.

2. CD-ROM directory is clicked.

3. Double click file the ABPM50_Setup.EXE.

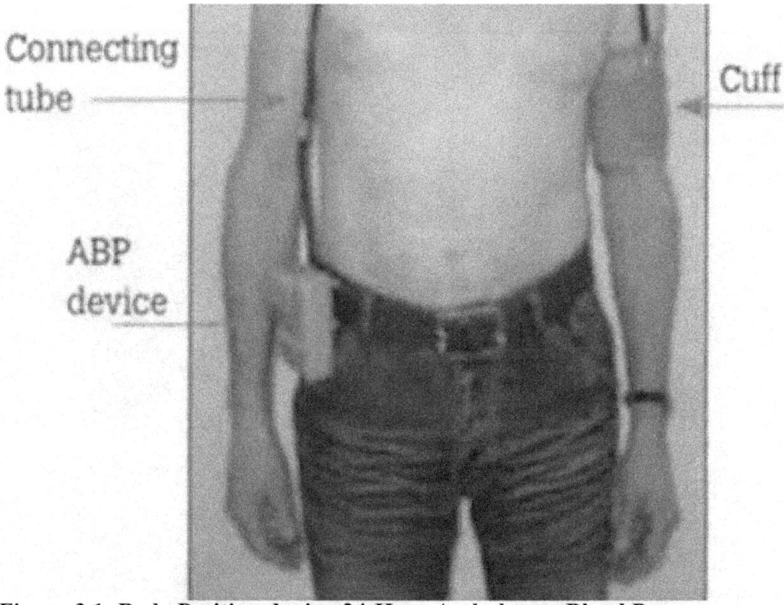

Figure-3.1: Body Position during 24-Hour Ambulatory Blood Pressure (ABPM)

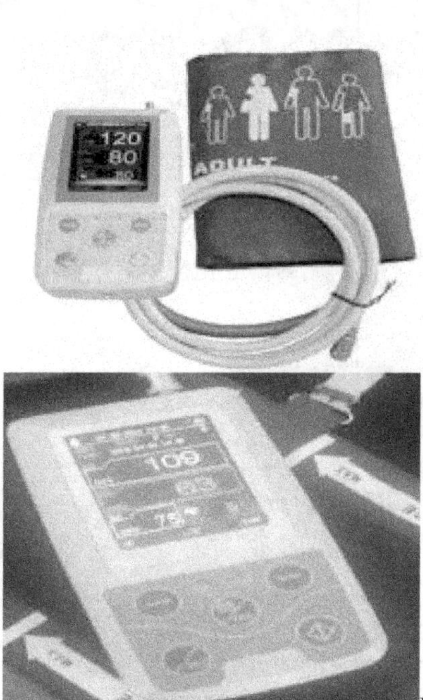

Figure-3.2: 24 Hours Ambulatory Blood Pressure Monitor

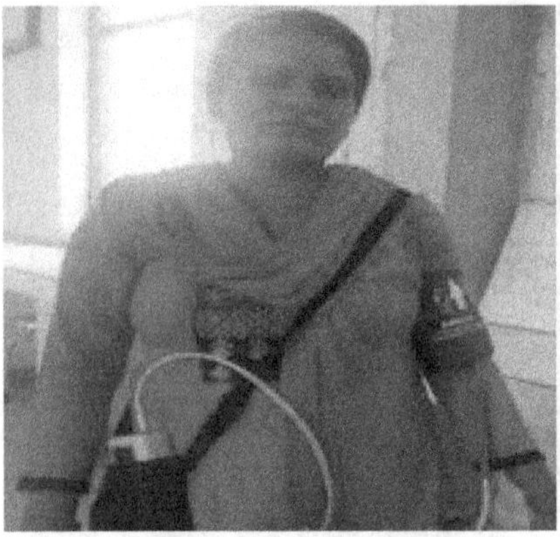
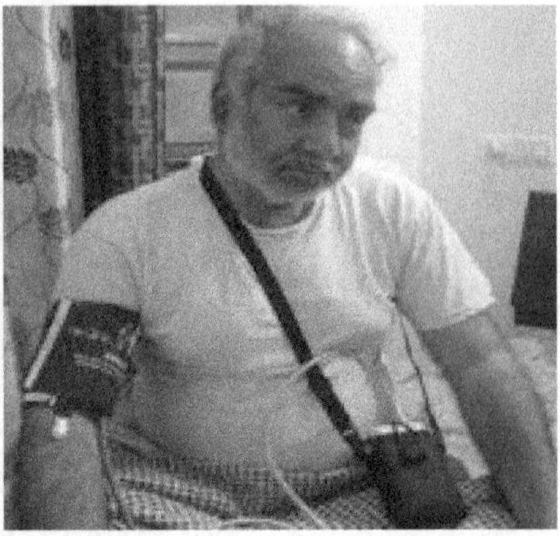
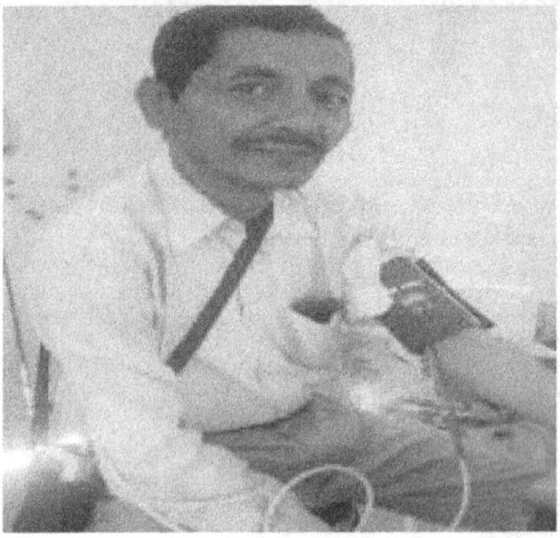
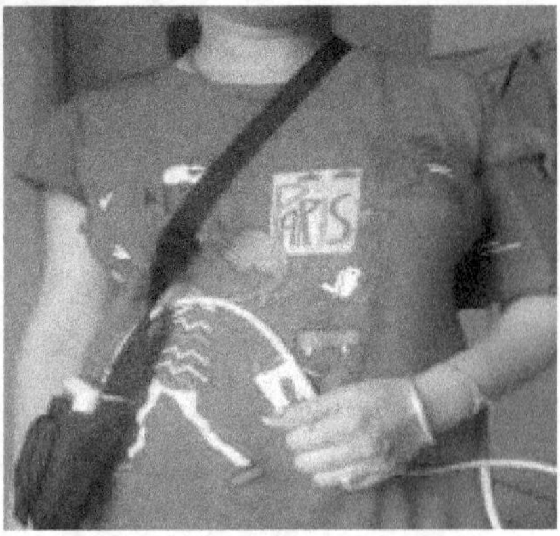
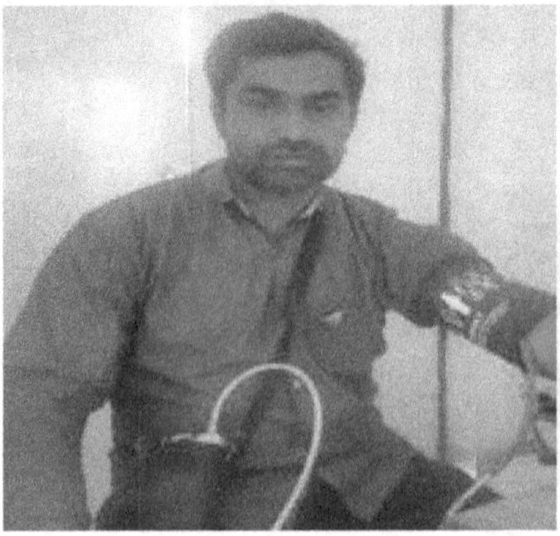
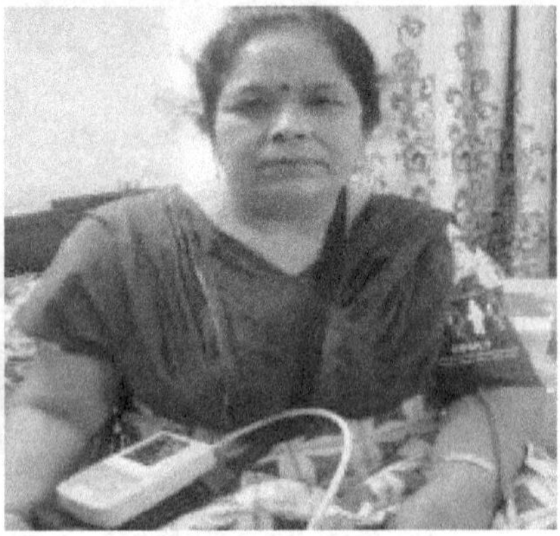

Figure-3.3(i): Measuring 24- Hours BP with ABPM CONTEC 50

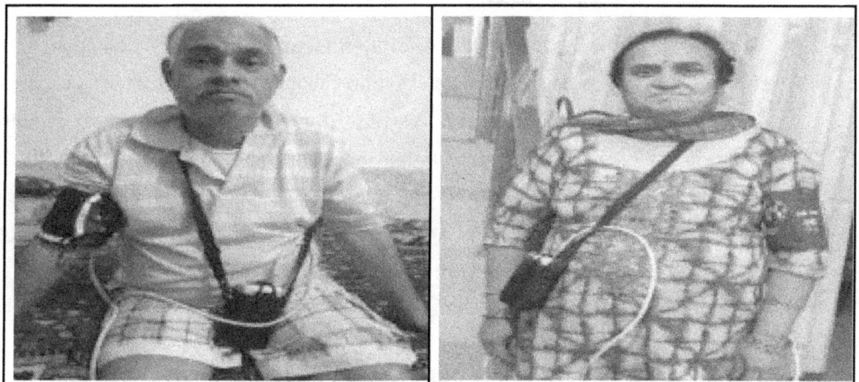

Figure-3.3(ii): Estimating 24- Hours BP during Routine Activities

STATISTICAL ANALYSIS

Data formed from BP & Pulse rate is examined by using particular A&D software. For computing a circadian rhythm Cosinor rhythmometry was used. By evaluating three components, i.e. Mesor, Amplitude and Acrophase, rhythms appear. For each variable, the rhythm detection ratio was analyzed. With the help of power spectrum process, prominent period (t) for each component was performed. This procedure is acceptable for both time series with the lost information and with non uniform time intervals data.

TESTS USED:

Tests were performed to see the differences in statistical components between different samples are due to sampling fluctuations or not.

1. CHI-SQUARE TEST: this test is applied when data is measured in attributes, i.e. during qualitative factors.

2. ANOVA (Analysis of variance)-F test: when there are more than two groups to be compared, analysis of variances is used in ANOVA, the variability of observations between &within the groups is taken into consideration. The overall variability is separated and test is applied.

3. REGRESSION: Means prediction, is use to detect the value of one character from other character. The variable to be estimated is dependent variables & which are known are independent variables.

4. t TEST: Is an statistical hypothesis test, which is used to compare the means of two groups.

5. Pearson's correlation: is used when we are finding linear relation among two variables.

SUBJECTS:

Randomly 180 normal individuals were selected; comprising of 90 women and 90 men and 120 unsystematically Hypertensive subjects were also taken, consisting of 45 Females and 75 males, who took part in our study.

Data was collected & analyzed, using ABPM during the years 2017 to 2019.The study was done in Panchkula, and the individuals were doing their day to day activities normally and didn"t claim any clinical issues.

DEMOGRAPHIC AND ANTHROPOMETRIC CHARACTERISTICS:

Several demographical i.e. age & sex and Anthropometrical components which includes body height (cm); body weight (kg); BSA (m2); and BMI (kg/m2) of every individual were taken. Smoking, alcohol drinking, intake of sleeping pills, Nature of work was asked & taken through questionnaires". During this current work duration, individuals were asked to note their sleeping time in their respective diaries, such as going to bed time, start of sleep time, and getting up time regularly.

All the included persons gave their written informed consent. The study got approval from Desh Bhagat University Ethics Committee.

COMPUTING BSA AND BMI OF HUMAN BODY:

Using DuBois method in 1916:

Surface Area of body (m^2) = 0.20247 x Height in m 0.725 x Weight in kg 0.425, the Surface Area of every person was computed by this method.

The Mass of body as

Mass Index (kg/m^2) = Weight in Kg divided by Height in m^2

EVALUATION OF BIORHYTHMS IN PRESSURE LEVEL AND PULSE RATE:

Using the device (ABPM, contec 50), day to day Pressure fluctuations of both SBP & DBP and Pulse Rate were calculated for at least 2-3 days in each subject. From these components, MAP and Rate pressure product were attained. During day (between 07:30 am -9:30 pm) BP components and HR were assessed every 20 min & in nighttime (between 9:40 pm - 07:10 am) every 40 min records were taken. Each one was requested to keep their arm unmoving while taking measurements. Full day subjects performed their day to day routine. After finished taking measurements, data was downloaded & analyzed in with the help of A&D application.

ABOUT MACHINE (ABPM contec-50):

The ABPM contec-50 measures a patient's blood pressure automatically, through twenty four-hours interval perfectly. ABPM50 is a computerized device.

It is based on oscillometric technique. It examines oscillometric measurements with blood running in arteria brachialis. With strap it can be wore, this has a plastic tube on one end & adult cuff, attached on the forelimbs.

BP COMPONENTS:

SBP: when the heart contracts, the pressure applied against the CVS. DBP: during rest, the pressure exerted against the cardiovascular system.

MAP: It is an average BP. It is formed from two components i.e. SBP & DBP readings (Drattsev et al., 2007).

$$MAP = DBP + [(SBP - DBP) / 3]$$

DP: It is also known as pressure rate product. It is used for detecting myocardial workload

$$DP = (SBP \times PULSE) / 100$$

HR: The number of time the heart beats in one minute.

NOCTURNAL BP DIPPING

Nightly BP dropping can be examined by the averages of day and nighttime BP. Based on night time dropping, individuals were arranged into three groups i.e. Extreme Dippers (Dipping more than 20%), Dippers (dipping lying between10% to 20%) and non-Dippers (dipping lying between 0% to 10%). Then Nightly dropping in every individual was examined by dipping method based on SBP (Kario *et al.*, 2000): (1 – nighttime SBP/daytime SBP)*100.

STATISTICAL INVESTIGATION:

Based on Age, Sex, Kind of duties and dropping style in BP Subjects were classified into different groups for analyzing details. Information formed for Pressure level and pulse rate was assessed using particular A&D application. Circadian rhythm in studied components was done by Cosinor rhythmometry. (Nelson et al., 1979).By three components, i.e. Mesor, Amplitude and Acrophase a rhythm & the rhythm detection proportion were calculated for every component. A power spectrum process was done for detecting prominent period in the time series for every component (De Prins *et al.*, 1986). By this procedure we get series of time with lost information and for non equivalent time interval data. Sex wise reliability in the spreading of nightly dropping was innovated by Chi-square test. Unidirectional analysis of variance followed by DMR test was done to notice the consequences of life span, kind of duties, and dropping style on biorhythm components. The t-test was petitioned to find out the statistically remarkable disputes between men and women in the means of all studied factors. With the help of Pearson correlations, Relationship of rhythm components of Systolic BP, Diastolic BP, MAP and pulse rate with demographical & anthropometrical factors, and sleeping features were also computed. With the SPSS (version 10), SPPC, CoStat (CoHort Software and Analysism ToolPak (Microsoft Excel), data was analyzed.

CHAPTER-IV

RESULTS AND DISCUSSION

TO STUDY AND DOCUMENTATION OF BLOOD PRESSURE AS WELL AS HEART RATE VARIABILITY IN NORMAL HUMANS FROM PANCHKULA, USING ABPM.

In normal individuals, we studied HR & BP Variability. Total 180 subjects were taken, out of which 90 were males and 90 females. Their demographical & anthropometrical features were calculated.

Table 4.1 Several Demographical & anthropometrical characteristics, and complete dipping in physically fit Normotensive males & females.

Sample size	**90 Males**	**90 Females**	**180 Both**
Body Weight (Kg)	64.80 ± 1.25	56.20 ± 1.21	60.03 ± 0.89
Body Height (cm)	168.78 ± 1.50	158.91 ± 0.78	163.40 ± 0.81
Surface Area of body (m^2)	1.71 ± 0.02	1.54 ± 0.02	1.62 ± 0.01
Mass Index of body (kg/m^2)	25.83 ± 0.45	24.86 ± 0.47	25.34 ± 0.33
Complete dipping in both	16.05 ± 0.80	16.61 ± 0.80	16.25 ± 0.60
Dipping in dippers	18.69 ± 0.51	18.23 ± 0.49	18.56 ± 0.43
Dipping in non-dippers	9.60 ± 0.49	9.17 ± 0.67	9.41 ± 0.39
Dipping in extreme dippers	27.07 ± 2.06	25.63 ± 1.25	26.06 ± 1.03

OCCURANCE OF DIPPERS, EXTREME DIPPERS AND NON-DIPPERS:

Total participants were 180 out of these 180 individuals 32 individuals were EDs, 90 were Ds and 58 were NDs (Fig 4.1 A). Both the factors i.e. Age as well as Dipping style are individualistic attributes exhibited by Chi-square results ($x^2 = 2.04$; df = 2; p = 0.36).

A: at group level

B. Males

Females

C.

Figure 4.1 Percentage prevalence: (A) at group level, (B) in Males (C) in Females of EDs, Ds and ND.

24

ALL COMPONENTS OF BP AND HR

RHYTHMIC DETECTION (RD):

A statistically remarkable biorhythm, calculated by a null hypothesis, was reported with respect to Age, Sex, type of work and dipping pattern for Systolic BP, Diastole BP, MAP, DP and Heart Rate components. The rhythmic proportion was more in young individuals but gradually declined with the growing age (Tab 4.2). In both Males and Females the rhythm detection ratio was considerably high. The rhythmic detective proportion in every component was increased in EDs as well as in Ds; although, NDs had fewer ratios in Systolic BP, Diastole BP and MAP with reference to dipping pattern (Tab 4.2).

Table 4.2 Illustrating RD ratio of BP components and Heart Rate with respect to Age, Sex and Dipping pattern.

Category		**Rhythm detection ratio**			
	Systol ic BP	**Diastol ic BP**	**Me an AP**	**Double Product**	**Heart Rate**
Age					
18-24	0.92	0.89	1.1	1.3	1.3

25-30	1.2	1.2	1	1.3	1
31-36	0.81	0.96	0.96	1.3	1.3
37-42	0.76	0.94	0.85	0.94	0.94
43-48	0.76	0.76	0.76	1.3	1.3
49-54	0.61	0.7	0.8	0.86	0.95
Gender					
Male (90)	0.85	0.87	0.84	1	1

Category		**Rhythm detection ratio**			
	Systolic BP	**Diastolic BP**	**Mean AP**	**Double Product**	**Heart Rate**
Female (90)	0.84	0.84	0.85	0.99	0.98
Dipping pattern					
Extreme dipper	1.3	1.3	1.3	1.3	1.3
Dipper	0.9	0.81	0.88	0.98	0.97
Non-dipper	0.72	0.89	0.78	1.3	1.3
All	0.83	0.85	0.84	1	0.99

Additionally, fig 4.2 (a-e) demonstrates the best-fitting cosine graphs in physically fit men & women at combined form of Systole BP, Diastole BP, MAP, DP, and HR. The curves in this said graph are formulated with the help of stats. With respect to Gender, curves indicate statistically significant biorhythms in Systole BP, Diastole BP, MAP, DP, and HR, (Fig 4.2 a-e). These graphs illustrate Mesor of Systole BP, Diastole BP, MAP and DP in males was high as compared to females (Fig 4.2 a-d). Nevertheless, in women"s the Mesor of HR was more than males (Fig 4.2 e).

a)

b)

c)

d)

e)

Figure 4.2 Normotensive Males and Females showing Cosine-fitted curves of (a) Systolic BP, (b) Diastolic BP, (c) MAP, (d) DP, and (e) HR.

Fig 4.3 (a-e) describes cosine graphs for Systole BP, Diastole BP, MAP, DP and HR irrespective of EDs, Ds and NDs at combined state. All three groups showed a statistically remarkable biorhythm in accordance to dipping pattern in Systole BP, Diastole BP, MAP, DP, and HR (Fig 4.3 a-e). Graph highlights that in ED, the Mesor of Systole BP, Diastole BP, MAP, DP, and HR were higher as compared to D and ND.

29

a)

b)

30

c)

d)

e)

Figure 4.3 Normotensive ED, D and ND at combined stage showing Cosine-fitted graphs of (a) Systolic BP, (b) Diastolic BP, (c) MAP, (d) DP, and (e) HR.

PERIOD:

Results shows that all the components i.e. Systole BP, Diastole BP, Mean AP, DP and pulse Rate are having 24h prominent phase in many individuals. In addition, frequency of prominent phase ($\tau = 24$ h or $\tau = 12$ h or $\tau \neq 24$ or $\tau \neq 12$ phase) of said components which results from power spectrum analysis is describe in Tab 4.3 (a-c) irrespective of Age, Gender and dipping style. According to our findings formulated by Chi-square test highlights that significant association was confirmed among Gender and prominent phase for Systolic BP only ($x^2 = 7.13$; df = 2; $p<0.05$) (Tab 4.3b).

Table 4.3(i) In accordance to Age the prevalence of prominent periods of BP components and HR.

Age Group	Prominent phase	Systolic BP	Diastolic BP	Mean AP	Double Product	Heart Rate
18 – 24	24 hrs	16	10	13	27	27
	12 hrs	11	16	12	5	4
	Other	8	9	11	3	4
25 – 30	24 hrs	19	18	18	21	22
	12 hrs	6	7	7	4	3
	Other	5	5	5	4	5
31 – 36	24 hrs	9	9	10	10	9
	12 hrs	5	4	4	4	3

	Other	4	5	4	4	7
37 – 42	24 hrs	7	6	6	8	9
	12 hrs	4	7	5	4	3
	Other	4	3	4	3	3
42 – 48	24 hrs	8	5	7	9	9
	12 hrs	4	5	5	3	3
	Other	3	5	3	3	3
49 – 54	24 hrs	6	6	6	6	7
	12 hrs	4	4	4	4	3
	Other	3	3	3	3	3

Table 4.3(ii) In accordance to Gender, prevalence of prominent periods of BP components and HR

Gender	**Prominent phase**	**Systolic BP**	**Diastolic BP**	**Mean AP**	**Double Product**	**Heart Rate**
Male	24 hrs	25	20	23	31	29
	12 hrs	10	10	10	6	4
	Other	6	11	8	4	8
Female	24 hrs	27	24	25	39	42
	12 hrs	13	18	15	6	3
	Other	9	7	9	4	4

Table 4.3(iii) In Accordance to Nocturnal Dipping Pattern, prevalence of Prominent Periods in Blood Pressure components and HR

Dipping pattern	Prominent phase	Systolic BP	Diastolic BP	Mean AP	Double Product	Heart Rate
Extreme dipper	24 hrs	7	7	8	11	11
	12 hrs	6	6	5	3	3
	Other	4	4	4	3	3
Dipper	24 hrs	35	30	33	44	44
	12 hrs	13	17	15	8	4
	Other	8	9	8	4	8
Non-dipper	24 hrs	12	10	10	18	19
	12 hrs	7	8	8	4	4
	Other	7	8	8	4	3
All	24 hrs	49	41	45	67	68
	12 hrs	20	25	22	9	4
	Other	12	15	14	5	9

However, significant relationship of age and nocturnal dipping with prominent periods of the studied components could not be confirmed (Table 4.3(i) and (iii)).

Figs 4.4-4.8 describes some of the samples of circadian as well as non-circadian prominent phase in BP components which includes Systole BP, Diastole BP, Mean AP, DP and pulse Rate biorhythms in single men, single women, single ED, D as well as single ND (Fig 4.8 a-e).Both men & women exhibited 24 hrs prominent phase in every elements (Figures 4.4 and 4.5). 24 h prominent period was also seen for BP components in extreme Dipper and Dipper (Figs 4.6 and 4.7). In Dipper 12 hrs small-scale subsidiary peak was also noticed in all components except HR (Fig 4.7). Twenty four hours regularity was revealed by Non-dippers in Systole BP, DP and pulse Rate (Fig 4.8 a, d & e). However, in the later, 16 h prominent period was found for DBP and Mean AP (Fig 4.8 b and c). Moreover, Tabs 4.4-4.8 present Amplitude and Acrophase for 24-h average, of Systolic BP, Diastolic BP, Mean AP,

DP and pulse Rate at combined stage irrespective of Age, Sex, type of duties and dipping style.

Period (τ)

Figure 4.4 Indicates prominent periods (τ) in healthy Normotensive males of all BP components i.e. Systolic BP (a), Diastolic BP (b), MAP (c), Double Product (d), and Heart Rate (e)

Figure 4.5 Demonstrative examples exhibiting prominent phase (τ) in healthy Normotensive females for all BP components i.e. Systolic BP (a), Diastolic BP (b), Mean AP (c), Double Product (d), and Heart Rate (e)

Figure 4.6 Several examples indicating prominent phase (τ) in an extreme dipper for various BP components i.e. Systolic BP (a), Diastolic BP (b), MAP (c), Double Product (d), and Heart Rate (e)

Figure 4.7 Various examples exhibiting prominent phase (τ) in dippers for various BP components i.e. Systolic BP (a), Diastolic BP (b), Mean AP (c), Double Product (d), and Heart Rate (e)

Figure 4.8 describing prominent phase (τ) in non-dippers for various BP components i.e Systolic BP (a), Diastolic BP (b), Mean AP (c), Double Product (d), and Heart Rate (e)

Circadian Mesor:

Systolic blood pressure (SBP): The findings of Cosinor rhythmometry shows twenty four hours inter-individual differences for Systolic BP. Least Circadian Mesor (112.82 ± 1.36 mm of Hg) was noticed in the age group 18-24 year and the highest (122.78 ± 3.68 mmHg) in 49-54 year irrespective of Age (Tab 4.4). Further, the Mesor was elevated in males (121.80± 1.39 mmHg) and decreased in a female which is about (111.32± 1.03 mmHg) (Tab 4.5). Based on type of work males do, the Mesor was maximum in day active workers (125.02 ± 1.80 mmHg) and the least (116.80 ± 4.39 mmHg) in night shift workers (Tab 4.6). Contrastingly women who were working had a more Mesor (115.39 ± 2.79 mmHg), but, was comparatively less in girls mainly students (108.39 ± 1.30 mmHg) (Tab 4.7). Additionally, based on dipping style the maximum day to day Mesor was seen in Extreme Dippers (124.30 ± 3.68 mmHg) after that Non-Dippers (118.06 ± 1.83 mm Hg) then finally Dippers (114.59 ± 1.37 mm Hg) (Tab 4.8).

One-way Analysis of variance accompanied by DMRT was appointed for discovering the outcomes of Age, work categories and dipping style on rhythms of Systole Blood Pressure. The t-test was conducted between males and females to test differences in rhythm parameters. Conclusions of both Analysis of variance as well as t-test are sum up in Tabular form in 2.4-2.8. Age showed no remarkable result on Mesor of Systole BP (Tab 4.4). A statistically significant differentiation between males and females was verified for Mesor of Systole BP ($p<0.001$) (Tab 4.5, Fig 4.10 a). It was found to be high in male when compared to females. Additionally, a remarkable outcome of type of work, disregarding of sex ($p<0.05$, $p<0.01$) and dropping style ($p<0.05$) were recorded for Systole BP (Tabs 4.6-4.8).

Table 4.4 According to Age**:** Circadian Mesor, Amplitude and Peak of BP components as well as HR

Components	**Age groups**				
	18 – 24	**25 – 30**	**31 – 36**	**37 – 42**	**43 – 48**
Mesor					

SBP	112.82 ± 1.36^{*,c}	116.92 ± 2.19^{bc}	117.77 ± 2.89^{abc}	115.73 ± 2.96^{bc}	120.24 ±
DBP	071.56 ± 0.78^{bc}	073.43 ± 1.13^{bc}	075.07 ± 1.38^{ab}	069.89 ± 2.06^{c}	075.37 ±
MAP	085.16 ± 0.92^{d}	087.33 ± 1.52^{dcd}	088.96 ± 1.94^{abc}	085.69 ± 2.21^{cd}	089.69 ±
DP	091.40 ± 1.75^{bc}	094.29 ± 2.13^{ab}	093.69 ± 2.59^{abc}	088.54 ± 3.65^{c}	097.80 ±
HR	082.31 ± 1.42^{a}	082.61 ± 1.23^{a}	081.88 ± 1.43^{a}	078.21 ± 2.50^{b}	083.09 ±
Amplitude					
SBP	12.13 ± 0.86^{bc}	13.17 ± 0.90^{ab}	14.81 ± 1.67^{a}	10.40 ± 1.47^{c}	11.83 ±
DBP	10.00 ± 0.55^{ab}	11.01 ± 0.53^{ab}	11.49 ± 1.03^{a}	09.28 ± 1.34^{b}	09.97 ±
MAP	10.56 ± 0.63^{abc}	11.32 ± 0.65^{ab}	12.32 ± 1.22^{a}	09.75 ± 1.25^{bc}	10.18 ±
DP	22.33 ± 1.18^{a}	23.57 ± 0.98^{a}	22.81 ± 1.64^{a}	20.37 ± 2.47^{a}	21.79 ±
HR	14.92 ± 0.80^{a}	14.86 ± 0.74^{a}	13.52 ± 0.81^{ab}	13.70 ± 1.66^{ab}	13.78 ±
Peak/Acrophase					
SBP	18.4 ± 0.2^{a}	18.4 ± 0.2^{a}	19.3 ± 0.5^{ab}	17.7 ± 0.9^{ab}	17.3 ±
DBP	18.4 0.2^{ab}	18.1 ± 0.3^{ab}	18.9 ± 0.4^{a}	17.3 ± 1.0^{b}	17.6
MAP	18.3 ± 0.2^{ab}	18.0 ± 0.3^{abc}	18.9 ± 0.5^{a}	17.2 ± 0.9^{c}	17.3
DP	18.4 ± 0.2^{ab}	18.6 ± 0.2^{ab}	18.9 ± 0.5^{a}	17.7 ± 0.8^{bc}	17.7
HR	18.6 ± 0.2^{a}	18.9 ± 0.2^{a}	18.8 ± 0.5^{a}	16.3 ± 1.1^{c}	18.1 ±

*Mean ± SE; Means having same superscripts didn't differ from one another at p 0.05 (on the basses of DMR test)41

Table 4.5 Circadian Mesor, Amplitude and Peak of BP components as well as Heart Rate according to sex-wise:

Components	Men	Women	t-value; degree of freedom; p
Mesor			
Systolic BP	121.80 ± 1.39	111.32 ± 1.03	08.90; 115; **<0.001**
Diastolic BP	075.55 ± 0.90	70.88 ± 0.68	07.25; 115; **<0.001**
Mean AP	90.69 ± 1.10	84.09 ± 0.80	08.16; 115; **<0.001**
DP	95.18 ± 1.70	91.29 ± 1.10	04.95; 115; < 0.06
Pulse Rate	79.74 ± 0.90	83.85 ± 0.95	07.16; 115; **<0.01**
Amplitude			
Systolic BP	12.68 ± 0.69	11.94 ± 0.70	03.76; 115; 0.47
Diastolic BP	10.40 ± 0.45	10.16 ± 0.51	03.33; 115; 0.35
Mean AP	10.86 ± 0.50	10.55 ± 0.58	03.40; 115; 0.68
DP	22.80 ± 0.99	21.08 ± 0.80	03.33; 115; 0.19
Pulse Rate	14.50 ± 0.59	13.91 ± 0.50	03.70; 115; 0.50
Peak			
Systolic BP	18.1 ± 0.5	18.2 ± 0.3	03.76; 115; 0.46
Diastolic BP	17.8 ± 0.4	18.2 ± 0.3	04.00; 115; 0.29
Mean AP	18.2 ± 0.4	18.1 ± 0.3	03.10; 115; 0.89
DP	18.2 ± 0.4	18.3 ± 0.3	03.92; 115; 0.35

Pulse Rate	18.4 ± 0.4	18.5 ± 0.4	03.60; 115; 0.59

Table 4.6 As a function of type of work in Male shift worker, male students & male day workers: Circadian Mesor, Amplitude and Acrophase of BP components and Heart Rate

Components	**Night Shift employees**	**School/college boys**	**Day active employees**	**Statistic value; degree of freedom; p**
Mesor				
Systolic BP	116.80 ± 4.39[*,a]	118.40 ± 2.38[a]	125.02 ± 1.80[a]	3.39; 2, 57; **<0.05**
Diastolic BP	74.00 ± 2.91[a]	74.29 ± 1.28[a]	76.66 ± 1.23[a]	3.98; 2, 57; 0.40
Mean AP	88.30 ± 3.29[a]	88.60 ± 1.68[a]	92.60 ± 1.40[a]	4.97; 2, 57; 0.16
DP	90.60 ± 5.36[a]	92.22 ± 2.94[a]	98.05 ± 2.15[a]	4.82; 2, 57; 0.19
Pulse Rate	78.88 ± 2.37[a]	79.49 ± 1.67[a]	80.10 ± 1.24[a]	3.20; 2, 57; 0.90
Amplitude				
Systolic BP	10.34 ± 1.59 [a]	14.12 ± 1.39 [a]	12.39 ± 0.89 [a]	4.47; 2, 57; 0.25
Diastolic BP	8.10 ± 1.19 [a]	11.22 ± 0.69 [b]	10.50 ± 0.59 [ab]	5.59; 2, 57; 0.09
Mean AP	8.62 ± 1.23 [a]	11.89 ± 0.90 [b]	10.79 ± 0.68 [ab]	5.20; 2, 57; 0.15
DP	19.89 ± 2.70 [a]	24.30 ± 1.70 [a]	21.61 ± 1.33 [a]	4.02; 2, 57; 0.40
Pulse Rate	13.19 ± 1.11 [a]	15.78 ± 1.28 [a]	14.03 ± 0.79 [a]	4.14; 2, 57; 0.38
Peak				
Systolic BP	19.2 ± 0.8 [a]	18.3 ± 0.4 [a]	17.3 ± 0.7 [a]	04.87; 2, 57; 0.17

Diastolic BP	18.6 ± 0.8 [a]	18.3 ± 0.4 [a]	17.8 ± 0.6 [a]	03.76; 2, 57; 0.47
Mean AP	18.5 ± 0.8[a]	18.1 ± 0.4 [a]	17.9 ± 0.6 [a]	03.69; 2, 57; 0.49
DP	19.0 ± 0.7 [a]	18.1 ± 0.3 [a]	17.9 ± 0.6 [a]	04.50; 2, 57; 0.23
Pulse Rate	18.8 ± 0.7 [a]	18.1 ± 0.4 [a]	17.8 ± 0.5 [a]	03.80; 2, 57; 0.46

Table 4.7 According to types of female work: Circadian Mesor, Amplitude and Peak of BP components and Heart Rate:

	House wives	**School/college girls**	**Working Ladies**	**statistic-value; degree of freedom; p**
Mesor				
Systolic BP	113.39 ± 1.97[*ab]	108.39 ± 1.30[a]	115.39 ± 2.79[b]	04.65; 2, 57; **<0.01**
Diastolic BP	70.08 ± 1.44[a]	70.20 ± 0.88[a]	73.94 ± 1.57[b]	02.89; 2, 57; 0.07
Mean AP	84.79 ± 1.48[ab]	82.57 ± 0.94[a]	86.80 ± 2.22[b]	02.72; 2, 57; 0.08
DP	90.60 ± 5.46[a]	91.89 ± 1.77[a]	91.70 ± 2.92[a]	00.34; 2, 57; 0.79
Pulse Rate	81.89 ± 1.58[a]	86.11 ± 1.54[a]	81.20 ± 1.67[a]	03.22; 2, 57; 0.053
Amplitude				
Systolic BP	11.71 ± 1.43[a]	11.40 ± 0.88[a]	13.66 ± 2.17[a]	00.86; 2, 57; 0.47
Diastolic BP	9.79 ± 1.06[a]	9.79 ± 0.74[a]	11.59 ± 1.39[a]	01.12; 2, 57; 0.37
Mean AP	10.41 ± 1.20[a]	10.19 ± 0.78[a]	11.48 ± 1.67[a]	00.47; 2, 57; 0.69
DP	20.60 ± 1.45[a]	21.38 ± 1.06[a]	20.96 ± 2.45[a]	00.21; 2, 57; 0.89

Pulse Rate	14.01 ± 1.17^{a}	14.47 ± 0.83^{a}	12.19 ± 1.03^{a}	01.44; 2, 57; 0.27
Peak				
Systolic BP	18.8 ± 0.6^{a}	18.4 ± 0.2^{a}	18.2 ± 0.4^{a}	00.63; 2, 57; 0.59
Diastolic BP	18.6 ± 0.4^{a}	18.3 ± 0.3^{a}	18.7 ± 0.6^{a}	00.26; 2, 57; 0.86
Mean AP	18.5 ± 0.5^{a}	17.8 ± 0.2^{a}	18.1 ± 0.3^{a}	00.57; 2, 57; 0.62
DP	18.8 ± 0.3^{a}	18.5 ± 0.2^{a}	18.1 ± 0.3^{a}	01.14; 2, 57; 0.36
Pulse Rate	18.1 ± 0.7^{a}	18.9 ± 0.2^{a}	18.2 ± 0.4^{a}	01.40; 2, 57; 0.28

Table 4.8 According to Dipping Pattern: Circadian Mesor, Amplitude and Peak of BP components and Heart Rate

Components		**Ds**	**NDs**	**Statistic value; degree of freedom; p**
Mesor				
SBP	$124.30 \pm 3.68^{*,a}$	114.59 ± 1.37^{b}	118.06 ± 1.83^{b}	04.35; 2,114; **<0.05**
DBP	78.05 ± 1.58^{a}	72.80 ± 0.80^{b}	72.66 ± 1.29^{b}	02.17; 2,114; 0.13
MAP	93.48 ± 2.23^{a}	86.39 ± 0.86^{b}	87.51 ± 1.45^{b}	03.43; 2,114; **<0.05**
DP	101.30 ± 3.67^{a}	92.26 ± 1.28^{b}	92.88 ± 2.09^{b}	02.43; 2,114; 0.10
HR	83.05 ± 1.46^{a}	82.30 ± 0.98^{a}	80.49 ± 1.39^{a}	00.87; 2,114; 0.46
Amplitude				
SBP	20.30 ± 1.70^{a}	12.58 ± 0.64^{b}	9.46 ± 0.81^{c}	23.32; 2,114; **<0.001**

DBP	14.22 ± 0.96^{a}	10.19 ± 0.51^{b}	9.28 ± 0.67^{b}	08.82; 2,114; **<0.001**
MAP	16.04 ± 1.15^{a}	11.10 ± 1.48^{b}	8.99 ± 0.69^{c}	14.93; 2,114; **<0.001**
DP	28.89 ± 1.34^{a}	21.58 ± 0.93^{b}	20.70 ± 1.07^{b}	10.21; 2,114; **<0.001**
HR	13.78 ± 0.84^{a}	13.90 ± 0.65^{a}	14.90 ± 0.81^{a}	00.80; 2,114; 0.49
Peak				
SBP	18.05 ± 0.54^{a}	17.88 ± 0.39^{a}	18.62 ± 0.50^{a}	01.20; 2,114; 0.33
DBP	18.03 ± 0.53^{a}	18.40 ± 0.34^{a}	17.80 ± 0.51^{a}	00.96; 2,114; 0.43
MAP	18.19 ± 0.49^{a}	18.09 ± 0.33^{a}	18.11 ± 0.51 ^{a}	00.13; 2,114; 0.99
DP	18.09 ± 0.51^{a}	18.09 ± 0.35^{a}	18.59 ± 0.32^{a}	00.92; 2,114; 0.46
HR	18.39 ± 0.56^{a}	18.19 ± 0.39^{a}	18.49 ± 0.32^{a}	00.29; 2,114; 0.82

DIASTOLE BLOOD PRESSURE:

DBP Circadian Mesor in the age categories 49-54 y (76.47 ± 2.80 mm of Hg) was highest and it was lowest in the age group 37-42 years (69.89 ± 2.00 mmHg) (Tab 4.4). Mesor was high in men (75.55 ± 0.90 mmHg) as compared to woman's (70.88 + 0.68 mmHg) (Tab 4.5). In Males according to type of work the Mesor was maximum in day active employees (76.66 ± 1.23 mmHg) and it was found to be the least in nightshift employees which was about (74.00 ± 2.91 mmHg) (Tab 4.6). However in Female subjects, in working women the Circadian Mesor was the highest (73.94 ± 1.57 mmHg) and less in house wife (70.08 ± 1.44 mmHg) (Tab 4.7). Moreover, Mesor was seen high in ED with reference to dipping pattern, (78.05 ± 1.58 mmHg) compared to Dippers (72.80 ± 0.80 mmHg) and ND (72.66 ± 1.29 mmHg) (Tab 4.8).

ANOVA outcomes highlights that none components, i.e. Age, type of work and dropping style performed remarkable effect on Mesor of Diastole BP (Tabs 4.4,

4.6-4.8). Nevertheless, a statistically significant (p<0.001) distinction was confirmed in males and females in the Mesor of the Diastolic BP. In males the Mesor of DBP significantly high when compared to subjects (Tab 4.5, Fig 4.9 b).

MEAN ARTERIAL PRESSURE:

Result indicates that with growing Age, the MAP rises (Tab 4.4). In the age group 18-24 year circadian Mesor was the lowest (85.16 ± 0.92 mmHg) and the highest (91.87 ± 2.95 mmHg) was found in age category 49-54 year. In males the Mesor was high (90.69± 1.10 mmHg) as compared to females (84.09 ± 0.80 mmHg) (Tab 4.5) irrespective of gender. According to type of work in males, the circadian Mesor was observed to be the highest in day active workers (92.60 ± 1.40 mmHg) and the lowest (88.30 ± 3.29 mmHg) in shift workers (Tab 4.6). In working women's, the circadian Mesor was highest (86.80 ± 2.22 mmHg) and in student it was lowest (82.57 ± 0.94 mmHg) (Tab 4.7). According to functions of dipping pattern the circadian Mesor in EDs was high (93.48 ± 2.23 mmHg) and in Ds it was low (86.39 ± 0.86 mmHg) (Tab 4.8).

Additionally, statistically significant cause of Age and work categories on Mesor of MAP couldn't be constructed (Tabs 4.4, 4.6-4.7). Satistically significant (p<0.001) difference was constructed in the Mesor of Mean AP in both males as well as in females. In males, Mesor of MAP was significantly higher as compared to females (Tab 4.5, Fig 4.9 C).

As a result, function of dipping pattern, when compared , ANOVA results indicated significant dipping cause on twenty four hours average of Mean AP (p<0.05). In EDs, Mean AP found to be more than NDs and Ds (Tab 4.8).

DOUBLE PRODUCT:

when subjects were compared Age-wised they gave maximum twenty four hours Mesor of DP among age categories 43-48 yrs (97.80 ± 2.89 mmHg) and least in the age range 37-42 yrs (88.54 ± 3.65 mmHg) (Tab 4.4). In male subjects the circadian Mesor was more (95.18 ± 1.70 mmHg) as compared to female subjects (91.29 ± 1.10 mmHg) (Tab 4.5). According to different work categories in men, the circadian Mesor found to be high in day active employees (98.05 ± 2.15 mmHg) and it was found to be low in nightshift employees (90.60 ± 5.36 mmHg) (Tab 4.6).Moreover in females work type, the circadian Mesor was the high in school/college going girls (91.89 ± 1.77 mmHg) and low in house wives (90.60 ± 5.46 mmHg) (Tab 4.7). In EDs circadian Mesor of DP was noticed high (101.30 ± 3.67 mmHg) and found low among Ds (92.26 ± 1.28 mmHg) (Tab 4.8).

Additionally, ANOVA outcomes point out that not even a single component i.e. age, variety of work and dipping style provided any significant cause on Mesor of DP (Tabs 4.4, 4.6-4.8). Similarly, in male subjects and female subjects significant differences couldn't be constructed among Mesor of DP, but in males, the range was increased (Tab 4.5, Fig 4.9 D).

HEART RATE:

The Mesor was noticed high among age range 43-48 yrs (83.09 ± 1.61 beats/ min) and low among 37-42 yrs age range (78.21 ± 2.50 beats/ min) (Tab 4.4). Additionally, in females Circadian Mesor (83.85 ± 0.95 beats/ min) was higher as compared to males (79.74 ± 0.90 beats/ min) (Tab 4.5). In day worker males the circadian Mesor was highest (80.08 ± 1.24 beats/ min) and the lowest in night shift employees (78.88 ± 2.37 beats/ min) (Tab 4.6). Likewise, in working women's the Mesor ranged between 81.20 ± 1.67 beats/ min to 86.11 ± 1.54 beats/ min in girls (Tab 4.7). According to dipping style, the Circadian Mesor was found to be elevated among EDs (83.05 ± 1.46 beats/ min) but NDs, it is found to be lowest (80.49 ± 1.39 beats/ min) (Tab 4.8). One-way ANOVA results illustrates that the Mesor was altered by the components, age, type of work and dipping pattern (Tabs 4.4, 4.6- 4.8). Moreover, in males & females a statistically significant difference ($p<0.01$) was constructed among Mesor. In females the Mesor was more in comparison to males (Tab 4.5, Fig 4.9 e).

CIRCADIAN AMPLITUDE:

Cosinor rhythmometry result shows inter-individual differences in circadian amplitudes in all the components, .i.e. Systolic BP, Diastole BP, MAP, DP and HR rhythms. As according to age, sex, type of work and dipping pattern. The circadian amplitudes of these rhythms at the group level are shown in Tabs 4.4-4.8.

SYSTOLIC BLOOD PRESSURE:

Age group subjects 31-36 year gives the highest amplitude (14.81 ± 1.67) and in the age group 49-54 amplitude was low (6.85 ± 1.72) (Tab 4.4). According to gender, in males, higher circadian amplitude was noticed (12.68± 0.69) as compared Women's (11.94 ±0.70) which ranges between 0.73 mmHg (Tab 4.5). In males, according to different duties, the circadian amplitude noticed in students was 14.12 ± 1.39 and 10.34 ± 1.59 in night shift employees (Tab 4.6). Moreover, in working ladies the amplitude was highest (13.66 ± 2.17) and in girls it was lowest (11.40 ± 0.88) (Tab 4.7). In addition, the circadian amplitude in extreme dippers was 20.30 ± 1.70 and in non dippers 9.46 ± 0.81 (Tab 4.8).

One-way ANOVA results states that, in every component only dipping style showed significant effect on amplitude of Systole BP (Tab 4.8). The results of DMR test guided by ANOVA for amplitude of Systolic BP are shown in the Fig 4.11. Amplitude was significantly increased in EDs as compared to Ds as well as NDs. Moreover, Ds had significantly more amplitude than NDs (Fig 4.11). Significant sex differences couldn't be constructed for amplitude of Systolic BP (Tab 4.5).

Figure 4.9 Comparison between males and females of circadian Mesors in all the components SBP (A), DBP (B), MAP (C), DP (D), and HR (E) in both males and females.** $p<0.01$, *** $p<0.001$, NS Not significant

DIASTOLIC BLOOD PRESSURE (DBP):

Individuals of age range between 31-35 yrs showed maximum amplitude (11.49 ± 1.03) while; the least amplitude (8.92 ± 1.41) was noticed in the age group 49-54 year (Tab 4.4). According to sex differentiation, circadian amplitude was more in males (10.40± 0.46) when compared to females (10.16 ± 0.51) which lie in between 0.23 mm of Hg (Tab 4.5). The school/college going boys had maximum amplitude (11.22 ± 0.69) and least (8.10 ± 1.19) was seen in nightshift employees (Tab 4.6). Additionally, the circadian amplitude was the maximum in working ladies (11.5 ± 1.39) and least in house wives (9.79 ± 1.06) (Tab 4.7). Now, based on dipping pattern, EDs showed maximum circadian amplitude (14.22 ± 0.96) and least was seen in NDs (9.28 ± 0.67). (Tab 4.8). Cause of parameters mainly age, variety of work as well as dipping pattern on amplitude of Diastolic BP were constructed by one-way ANOVA. Outcomes indicate that only dipping pattern gave significant effect on amplitude (Tab 4.8). Amplitude in EDs was statistically significantly more as compared to Ds as well as NDs (Tab 4.8, Fig 4.10). Moreover, significant differences couldn't be constructed for circadian amplitude with reference to sex (Tab 4.5).

MEAN ARTERIAL PRESSURE (MAP):

In age range 31-36 yrs the circadian amplitude of MAP was found to be maximum (12.32 ± 1.22) and least (8.95 ± 1.50) in 49-54 yrs (Tab 4.4). Males showed more circadian amplitude (10.86 ± 0.50) as compared to females (10.55 ± 0.58) (Tab 4.5). According to work differentiation in males, the circadian amplitudes was noticed between 8.62 ± 1.23 in nightshift employees and 11.89 ± 0.90 in school/college going boys (Tab 4.6). Moreover, in females, the amplitude was more in working ladies (11.48 ± 1.67) and least in school/college going girls (10.19 ± 0.78) (Tab 4.7). Additionally, EDs produced high amplitude (16.01 ± 1.05) and least was seen in NDs (8.99 ± 0.69). It had a range of 10.04 mmHg (Tab 4.8).

Findings of one-way ANOVA explain statistically significant effect of dipping style on amplitude (Tab 4.8). For amplitude, outcomes of DMR test followed the ANOVA

which are shown in the Fig 4.11. In EDS Amplitude was significantly high in comparison to DS and NDs. however, Ds had significantly high amplitude as than NDs (Fig 4.11).

On amplitude both age and types of duties didn't exhibited any significant effect (Tabs 4.4 & 4.6-4.7). No difference was seen to be significant according to sex wise (Tab 4.5).

DOUBLE PRODUCT:

In age group 25-30 yrs, circadian amplitude was highest (23.57 ± 0.98) and least (17.04 ± 1.87) in age range 49-54 yrs. The amplitude had a range of 9.53 mmHg, regardless of age (Tab 4.4). According to sex, in males, circadian amplitude was maximum (22.80 ± 0.99) as compared to females (21.08 ± 0.80) which lies in between 1.7 mmHg (Tab 4.5). According to type of work, the circadian amplitude was seen 19.89 ± 2.70 in male nightshift employees and 24.30 ± 1.70 in school/college going boys (Tab 4.6). As in school/college girls circadian amplitude was maximum (21.42 ± 0.96) and least in house wives (20.59 ± 1.35) (Tab 4.7).Additionally, in EDs the high circadian amplitude (28.90 ± 1.24) and least in NDs (20.67 ± 0.97) with a range of 11.23 mmHg (Tab 4.8).

One-way ANOVA results illustrates that age didn't have any significant result on DP amplitude. Moreover, outcomes of DMR test signify that the amplitude dropped in old aged persons in comparison to young individuals (Tab 4.4).

There was no significant difference in the amplitude of the DP among males as well as females (Tab 4.5). In both males and females, work type was not significant on amplitude of DP (Tab 4.6-4.7). Accordingly, when they were compared according to dipping patterns, findings of ANOVA gave significant ($p<0.001$) dipping effect on amplitude of DP. Amplitude was statistically significantly more in EDs in comparison to Ds as well as NDs (Tab 4.8, Fig 4.10).

HEART RATE:

In accordance to age the maximum circadian amplitude (14.92 ± 0.80) was seen in individuals of age gp 18-24 yrs and least (11.95 ± 1.28) in 49-54 yrs (Tab 4.4). According to sex wise, males had high circadian amplitude (14.50 ± 0.60) in comparison to females (13.91 ± 0.50) (Tab 4.5). Categorization of individuals in accordance to type of work in males revealed maximum circadian amplitude (15.78 ± 1.28) in school/college going boys and least

(13.19 ± 1.11) in nightshift employees (Tab 4.6). Likewise, in females, the school/college going girls had maximum circadian amplitude (14.47 ± 0.83) and least (12.19 ± 1.03) was seen in working ladies (Tab 4.7). Additionally, maximum circadian amplitude was seen in NDs (14.90 ± 0.81) and least in EDs (13.78 ± 0.84 (Tab 4.8).

Excitingly, outcomes of ANOVA described that no factors showed any significant result on amplitude of HR (Tabs 4.4, 4.6-4.8). Difference for amplitude was also not signified among males and females (Tab 4.5). Findings of DMR test followed the

ANOVA, as function of dipping pattern for amplitude of HR is shown in the Fig 4.10.

Figure 4.10 Comparison of Circadian Amplitude according to Dipping Pattern of Systolic BP, Diastolic BP, Mean AP, Double P and Heart Rate. The means have same alphabets are not statistically significant from one another at $p<0.05$ among different groups for individual variable (on the basis of DMR test).

CIRCADIAN PEAK /ACROPHASE:

The results of Cosinor rhythmometry indicated inter-individual differences in the level of acrophase of SBP, DBP, MAP, DP and HR. At the group level the circadian acrophases of these rhythms are presented in Tabs 4.4-4.8 as function of age, sex wise, work type and dipping pattern.

SYSTOLIC BLOOD PRESSURE:

Alteration in circadian peak of Systolic BP was also observed at combined stage. Moreover, the average peak of the systolic BP arrived mainly in the afternoon, regardless of age, sex wise, type of duties and dipping pattern (Tabs 4.4-4.8). The peak spread for Systolic BP was 2.3 h in normal individuals when differentiated among various groups as per age. The peak arrived at the earliest (14.0 h) in the age range 49-54 year and at the latest (16.3) in the age range 31-36 year (Tab 4.4). According to sex wise, the peak time appeared more constant stable as spread of only 0.3 h. Peak appeared at 18.1 h in males and 18.2 h in females, (Tab 4.5). Additionally, peak arrived at 19.2 h in male nightshift employees and 17.3 h in day active males with a spread of 5.0 h (Tab 4.6).

The peak of Systolic BP biorhythm appeared among 18.2 h in working ladies and 18.8 h in house wives with a spread of only 3.7 h (Tab 4.7). Further, the earliest peak appeared in Ds (17.88 h) and latest (18.62 h) in NDs. The peak spread was 3.7 h (Tab 4.8). ANOVA results shows that the parameters like age, type of duties and dipping style didn't gave any significant effect on peak of Systolic BP (Tabs 4.4, 4.6-4.8). Moreover, peak appeared earlier in old age peoples as compared to young population (Tab 4.4). Significant difference couldn't be constructed among males and females (Tab 4.5).

DIASTOLIC BLOOD PRESSURE:

Alterations in circadian peak of Diastolic BP were seen at combined stage. The peak of Diastolic BP biorhythm appeared at 17.3 h (in the age range 37-42 year) and 18.9 h (in the age range 31-36 year). The spread for Diastolic BP was 4.6 h (Tab

4.4). Peak appeared at 17.8 h in males and 18.2 h in females (Tab 4.5). According to types of duties in males, the peak appeared at 17.8 h in day active employees, whereas it occurred at 18.6 h in nightshift employees and 18.3 h in school/college boys with a spread of 3.8 h (Tab 4.6). According to work differentiation in females the peak arrived at the earliest (18.3 h) in girls and the latest (18.6 h) in house wives and working ladies with a stable spread of 3.3 h (Tab 4.7).

When the individuals were differentiated according to dipping style, the earliest peak arrived in NDs (17.7 h) and the latest (18.3) in Ds. The peak spread was 3.6 h (Tab 4.8). Additionally, ANOVA outcomes didn't produced any significant result of age, type of duties and dipping style on peak of Diastolic BP (Tabs 4.4, 4.6-4.8). Further, advancement in peak was also seen with the growing age (Tab 4.4). Significant difference couldn't be represented among males and females (Tab 4.5).

MEAN ARTERIAL PRESSURE (MAP):

Alterations in Circadian peak of MAP were also seen at combined stage. The peak appeared at the earliest (17.2 h) in age group 37-42 year and at the latest (18.9 h) in the age group 31-36 year (Tab 4.4). The peak spread for MAP was 4.7 h. According to sex, the peak timings appeared with a stable spread of 3.1 h. In males, peak appeared at 18.2 h and in females it was 18.1 h (Tab 4.5).

Additionally, the peak of MAP biorhythm arrived between 17.9 h in day actives and 18.5 h in night shift employees) with a spread of 4.1 h (Tab 4.6). according to varies duties in females, the peak appeared at the earliest (17.8 h) in girls and the latest

(18.5 h) in house wives with a spread of 3.4 h only (Tab 4.7). According to dipping pattern, the earliest peak (18.11 h) appeared in NDs and the latest (18.09 h) in Ds and EDs. The peak spread was 3.1 h only (Table 4.8). Results of ANOVA showed that none of the factors, such as age, work type and dipping pattern gave any significant effect on peak of MAP (Tabs 4.4, 4.6-4.8). Further, sex wise difference for peak of MAP was not significant (Tab 4.8).

DOUBLE PRODUCT (DP):

Difference in circadian peak of DP was also noticed at combined stage. According to age, the peak appeared at the earliest (17.2 h) in the age 49-54 year and at the latest (18.9 h) in the age 31-36 year. The peak spread was 4.7 h (Tab 4.4). According to sex, the peak timings arrived with a spread of 3.3 h only. The peak appeared at 18.2 h in males and 18.3 h in females (Tab 4.5). The peak timings occurred with a spread equal to 4.4 h when the male were differentiated on the basis of various works. The peak of DP biorhythm arrived among 17.9 hrs in day active employees and 19.0 h in nightshift employees (Tab 4.6). In women's, the peak arrived at the earliest (18.1 h) in working ladies and the latest (18.8 h) in house wives with a spread of 3.7 h (Tab 4.7). According to dipping style, that the earliest peak (18.09 h) arrived in both EDs as well as in Ds and the latest (18.59 h) in NDs with a peak spread of 3.5 h (Tab 4.8).

Results of ANOVA showed a statistically significant ($p<0.05$) effect of age on peak of DP biorhythm. In old aged, statistically significant advancement in peak was apparent when compared with young individuals (Tab 4.4). Moreover, peak of DP wasn't influenced by various parameters, like type of duties they perform and dipping pattern (Tabs 4.6-4.8). Comparison among peak of males and females didn't lead to rejection of the null hypothesis (Tab 4.5).

HEART RATE (HR):

Alterations in Circadian peak of HR biorhythm was also seen at combined stage when individuals were differentiated into various groups, based on age, sex, type o work and dipping style. The peak spread for HR biorhythm was 5.6 h in Normal individuals as per age. The peak appeared at the earliest (16.3 h) in the age 39-42 year and latest (18.9 h) in the age 25-30 year (Tab 4.4). According to sex, the peak time occurred with a spread of 3.2 h only. Peak appeared at 18.4 h in males, whereas in female its 18.5 h (Tab 4.5). Moreover, the earliest peak (17.8 h) was seen in day active and latest (18.8 h) in nightshift employees with a spread of 4.0 h. In the house wives, the peak appeared at the earliest (18.1 h) and the latest (18.9 h) in girls with a spread equal to 3.8 h. According to dipping pattern, the earliest it arrived in

Ds (18.19 h) and the latest (18.49 h) in the NDs. The peak spread was 3.3 h only (Tab 4.8).

One-way ANOVA outcomes explains a statistically significant ($p<0.01$) result of age on peak of HR biorhythm. A statistically significant advancement in peak was constructed with growing age (Tab 4.4). Components type of work and dipping style didn't gave any significant result on DP (Tabs 4.6-4.8). Significant difference was also not constructed among peaks of males and females (Tab 4.5).

CORRELATION OF BIORHYTHM SIGNIFICANCE OF BP COMPONENTS & HR AMONG DEMOGRAPHICAL & ANTHROPOMETRICAL ELEMENTS AND SLEEP PARAMETERS

Tab 4.9 Shows relationship of age, height, weight, Surface Area, Mass Index of body, sleeping time, wakening time, and sleep duration of individuals with biorhythm elements of Systolic BP, Diastolic BP, MAP, DP and PR. Outcomes reveals less pairs of components showed significant relationship among one another. 24-h average of HR was significantly positively related with Mass Index of body ($p<0.05$).

A statistically significant negative connection was constructed among amplitude of Systolic BP and BMI ($p<0.05$). Similarly amplitude of MAP was significantly negatively related with weight ($p<0.01$) and Surface Area ($p<0.01$). Amplitude of HR gave significant negative relation with weight ($p<0.05$) and positive relation with sleeping time ($p<0.05$). Additionally, peak of Diastolic BP exhibited significant negative relation with BMI ($p<0.05$) and positive connection with sleep duration ($p<0.05$). Moreover, DP didn't show any significant connection with demographical or anthropometrical components or sleep elements (Tab 4.9).

Table 4.9 Rhythm Correlations with Demographical & Anthropometrical elements, and sleeping parameters of BP components and Heart Rate at group level

Components	Systolic BP	Diastolic I		Double Product	Heart Rate
Mesor					
Age	.054†	-.118	-.029	.019	.061
Height	.183	.117	-.057	.189	.108
Weight	-.035	-.054	-.111	-.033	-.137
Surface Area	.056	.018	-.110	.060	-.072
BMI	-.148	-.118	-.074	-.149	.101*
Awakening time	-.030	-.038	.032	-.048	.016
Sleeping time	-.041	.017	.080	-.052	.050
Sleep duration	-.020	.045	.057	-.013	.043
Amplitude					
Age	-.071	-.077	-.055	-.043	-.014
Height	-.050	-.121	-.169	-.039	-.073
Weight	-.059	-.138	-.251**	-.012	-.204*
Surface Area	-.056	-.149	-.262**	-.017	-.184
BMI	-.029*	-.081	-.191	.034	-.186
Awakening time	.075	.050	.096	.082	.091
Sleeping time	.164	.176	.119	.165	.199*
Sleep duration	.095	.131	.030	.090	.113
Peak					

Age	-.172	.023	.077	-.154	-.075
Height	-.192	.065	-.182	.016	-.185
Weight	-.156	-.145	.095	-.157	-.163
Surface Area	-.189	-.097	.143	-.114	-.192
BMI	-.066	-.198*	-.012	-.177	-.087
Awakening time	-.060	-.180	-.080	-.050	-.019
Sleeping time	-.049	.054	.092	.110	-.066
Sleep duration	.22	.220*	.158	.147	-.055

‡Pearson's correlation coefficient, *p<0.05, **p<0.01

DIURNAL & NOCTURNAL BLOOD PRESSURE AND HEART RATE IN NORMAL HUMANS FROM PANCHKULA

DIURNAL & NOCTURNAL AVERAGES OF VARIABLES OF BP AND HEART RATE ACCORDING TO SEX: Tab 4.10 shows the ranges of various BP components and HR in day and night according to sex. The information was collected with the help of the A&D software from every one. Outcomes of t-test implifies that averages of Systolic BP, Diastolic BP, and MAP were significantly more in male subjects as compared to female subjects (p<0.01, p<0.001), regardless of time, i.e., diurnal & nocturnal. Moreover, in females average of HR was significantly high when compared with males, regardless of time (p<0.01) (Tab 4.10).

Table 4.10 Comparison according to gender of averages for BP components and HR formed in day and night in normotensive subjects

Components	Males	Females	Both	t-value; df; p
Diurnal				

SBP(mmHg)	124.35 ± 1.58	116.63 ± 1.23	121.49 ± 1.13	5.44; 115; **<0.001**
DBP(mmHg)	079.56 ± 0.94	075.14 ± 0.84	077.35 ± 0.69	4.05; 115; **<0.001**
	) 094.85 ±	088.73 ± 0.94	091.79 ± 0.82	4.74; 115; **<0.001**
HR(mmHg)	084.89 ± 1.08	089.31 ± 1.09	087.10 ± 0.83	3.26; 115; **<0.01**
Nocturnal				
SBP(mmHg)	110.54 ± 1.55	101.08 ± 1.19	105.81 ± 1.10	5.27; 115; **<0.001**
DBP(mmHg)	067.40 ± 1.26	062.87 ± 0.98	068.14 ± 0.95	3.21; 115; **<0.01**
	) 081.17 ±	074.86 ± 0.88	078.01 ± 0.86	4.56; 115; **<0.001**
HR(mmHg)	069.49 ± 1.16	074.37 ± 1.26	071.93 ± 0.92	3.20; 115; **<0.01**

EFFECT OF AGE, TIME, SEX, AND DIPPING PATTERN ON BP COMPONENTS AND HEART RATE

Tab 4.11 shows sum up of two-way ANOVA that was indicating to compute the effects of age (6 groups) and time (daytime vs. nighttime). Both the factors produced a statistically significant effect on Systole BP (age: $p<0.01$; time: $p<0.001$) and Mean Arterial Pressure (age: $p<0.01$; time: $p<0.001$).

In addition, unconventional effect of time was constructed on Diastole BP ($p<0.001$) and Heart Rate ($p<0.001$). Nevertheless, no connection effects are significant (Tab 4.11).

Table 4.11 Age effect (6 groups of age) and time duration (T) on BP components as well as Heart Rate by Two-way

Components	Factors	Sum of Square	Degree of freedom	Mean Square	Statistic	P

Systolic BP	Age	2250.54	5, 219	690.10	13.48	**<0.01**
	Time duration	14243.37	1, 219	14243.37	134.63	**<0.001**
	Age x Time	856.57	5, 219	411.31	10.99	0.43
Diastolic BP	Age	663.37	5, 219	372.67	11.41	0.23
	Time duration	8798.52	1, 219	8798.52	175.7	**<0.001**
	Age x Time	766.89	5, 219	393.37	11.82	0.12
MAP	Age	1062.61	5, 219	452.52	12.51	**<0.01**
	Time duration	11124.74	1, 219	11124.74	188.14	**<0.001**
	Age x Time	558.59	5, 219	351.71	01.85	0.52
Pulse Rate	Age	672.92	5, 219	374.58	02.10	0.37
	Time duration	13426.75	1, 219	13426.75	194.84	**<0.001**
	Age x Time	693.99	5, 219	378.79	11.16	0.34

Additionally, Tab 4.12 illustrates the effects of sex wise in both males as well as in females and time during day as well as in night on all BP components. Outcomes derives a statistically significant cause of both the factors on Systole BP ($p<0.001$), DBP ($p<0.001$), MAP ($p<0.001$), and HR (sex: $p<0.01$; time: $p<0.001$). A

connection of these factors also provides significant result on Systole BP only (Tab 4.12).

Table 4.12 Effects of Sex wise (S) and time duration (T) on BP components As well as on Heart Rate by Two-way ANOVA:

Component			Degree of freedom	Mean Sq	Statistic	P
Systolic BP	Sex	3940.00	1, 227	3940.00	045.44	**<0.001**
	Time duration	14306.00	1, 227	14306.00	146.39	**<0.001**
	S x T	470.21	1, 227	470.21	11.65	**<0.001**
Diastolic BP	Sex	991.26	1, 127	991.26	023.90	**<0.001**
	Time duration	8761.93	1, 127	8761.93	180.18	**<0.001**
	S x T	58.00	1, 127	58.00	1.12	0.29
MAP	Sex	1621.93	1, 127	1621.93	033.27	**<0.001**
	Time duration	11042.21	1, 127	11042.21	199.17	**<0.001**
	S x T	413.68	1, 127	413.68	03.00	0.16
Heart Rate	Sex	1454.25	1, 127	1454.25	027.84	**<0.01**
	Time duration	13594.21	1, 127	13594.21	215.53	**<0.001**
	S x T	0.84	1, 127	0.76	0.01	0.91

Tab 4.13 indicates nightly dipping style in EDs as well as in Ds and in NDs as well and time in day as well as in night on these said factors. Statistically significant independent effects of both the factors was constructed on Systole BP ($p<0.01$), Diastole BP ($p<0.01$), and MAP ($p<0.001$). In HR, the effect of time was seen significant ($p<0.001$). Connections of these variables also provided significant

effects on every said variables excluding Pulse Rate (Tab 4.13).

Table 4.13 Effects of night time dipping Pattern (NDP) and time duration (T) on BP components as well as in Heart Rate by Two-way ANOVA:

	Sum of Sq		**Degree of freedom**	**Mean Sq**	**Statistic**	**P**
Systolic BP	Night DP	2611.30	2, 225	1455.65	021.28	**<0.01**
	Time	14940.03		14940.03	153.02	**<0.01**
	Night DP x T	2746.20	2, 225	1523.10	021.94	**<0.01**
Diastolic		806.75	2, 225	553.37	15.26	**<0.01**
	Time	8798.52	1, 225	8798.52	186.65	**<0.01**
	Night DP x T	1016.86	2, 225	658.43	08.45	**<0.01**
MAP	Night DP	1178.90	2, 225	739.45	08.80	**<0.001**
	Time	10987.37		10987.37	199.69	**<0.001**
	Night DP x T	1475.28	2, 225	887.64	11.43	**<0.001**
Heart Rate	Night DP	4747.20	2, 225	2473.60	2183.60	0.70
	Time	26326.73		26326.73	12.930	**<0.001**
	Night DP x T	4002.26	2, 225	1151.13	0.948	0.43

Findings of DMR test followed the ANOVA for Systolic BP, Diastolic BP, Mean AP, and Pulse Rate are shown in Fig 4.11 (a-d). Diurnal Systolic BP, Diastolic BP, and Mean AP were significantly elevated in EDs in comparison to Ds and NDs. Moreover, nocturnal Systolic BP, Diastolic BP, and Mean AP were significantly increased in NDs when compared to Ds and EDs (Fig 4.11 a-c).

Additionally, EDs showed significantly more nocturnal Mean AP in comparison to Ds (Fig 4.11 c). When seen in HR significant differences couldn't be constructed in Ds, NDs, as well as in EDs, regardless of time (Fig 4.11 d).

CORELATION OF DAY & NIGHTLY BP COMPONENTS AS WELL AS HEART RATE WITH DEMOGRAPHICAL & ANTHROPOMETRICAL PARAMETERS, AND SLEEP ELEMENTS

Pearson's correlation coefficients of day and night with demographical & anthropometrical parameters such as age, body height, body weight, Surface Area and Mass Index of body) and sleep elements (wakening time, sleeping time and sleep duration) Systolic BP, Diastolic BP, Mean AP, and Pulse R at combined stage, in accordance to sex and dipping pattern are presented in Tabs 4.14, 4.15 & 4.16, respectively.

An outcome signifies that Systole BP was statistically significantly positively related to Age, Body Height, Body Weight, Surface Area and Mass Index of body, regardless of time. The diurnal Diastole BP revealed significant +ve connection with body weight, Surface Area and Mass Index, and nocturnal Diastole BP indicates +ve correlation with respect to Age, body weight, Surface Area and Mass Index. During daytime and nightly, MAP revealed statistically significant +ve relationship with height, weight, Surface Area and Mass Index. Moreover in night, MAP also express +ve relation with age. In addition, with respect to weight and BSA during daytime Heart Rate showed significant negative relationship and positive relationship with BMI. Irrespective of the time HR also recorded positive association with sleep length, however, with sleep parameters, significant connected of Systolic BP, Diastolic BP and MAP couldn't be constructed (Tab 4.14).

Table 4.14 Demographic & Anthropometric variables, and sleep parameters of BP components and HR at group level with Correlation of Daytime and night time.

Components		**Diastolic BP**	**MAP**	**Heart Rate**
		DIURNAL		
Age	.228*,†	.137	.186	-.165
Height	.202*	.168	.195*	-.123
Weight	.345**	.288**	.297**	-.251**
Surface Area	.336**	.277**	.297**	-.241*
BMI	.273**	.229*	.224*	.216*
Awakening time	.036	.103	.081	.084
Sleeping time	-.165	-.061	-.125	.149
Sleep duration	-.186	-.151	-.192	.218*
		NOCTURNAL		
Age	.341**	.237*	.282**	-.003
Height	.256**	.109	.244*	-.101
Weight	.358**	.287**	.360**	-.053
Surface Area	.366**	.254**	.361**	-.085
BMI	.246*	.250*	.255**	.004
Awakening time	.018	.075	.080	-.089
Sleeping time	-.114	-.079	-.100	.103

Sleep duration	-.119	-.141	-.166	.198*

Pearson's correlation coefficient, *p<0.05, **p<0.01

Additionally, Tab 4.15 represents relationship among pair of factors in accordance to Sex wise. Outcomes reveal that in men's, significant correlation couldn't be constructed in day between any one pair. Moreover, in women's, diurnal Systolic BP and Mean AP displayed significant +ve relation with weight and BMI. A significant

CPSIA information can be obtained
at www.ICGtesting.com
Printed in the USA
LVHW080004061222
734629LV00016B/1273